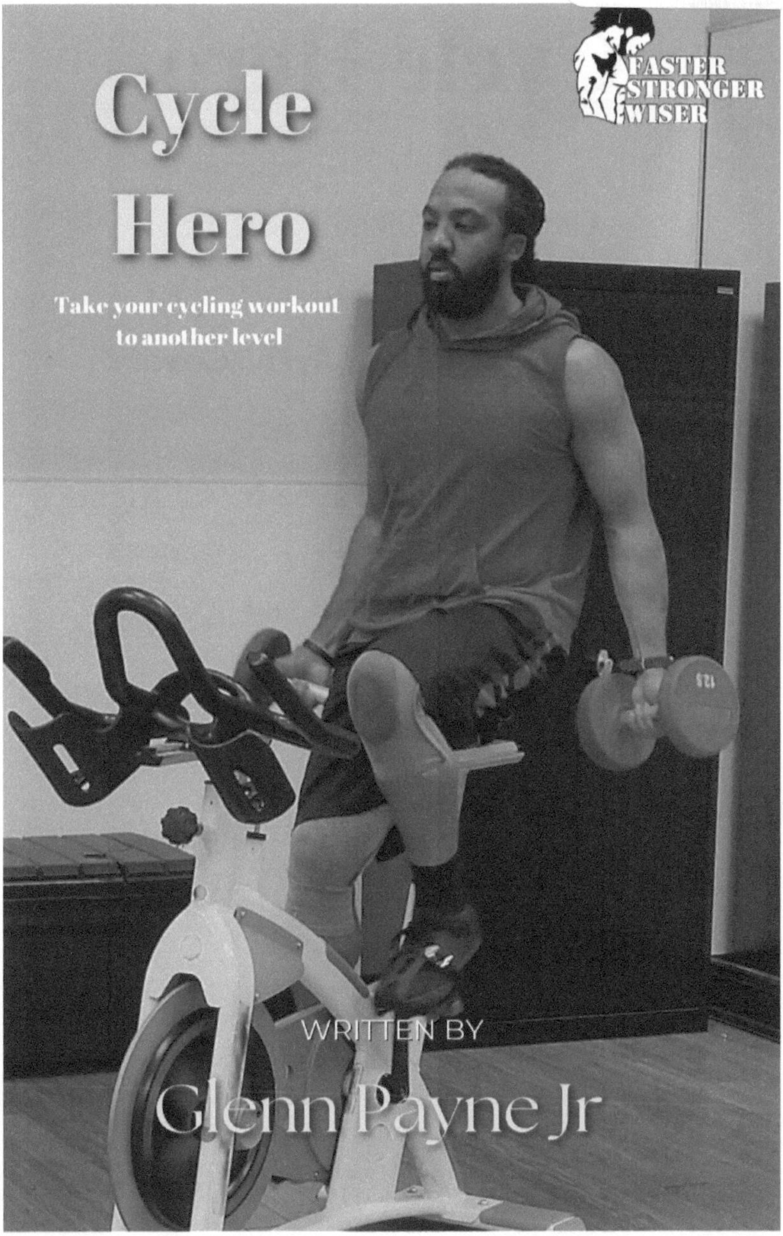

Cycle Hero

Take your cycling workout to another level

FASTER STRONGER WISER

WRITTEN BY

Glenn Payne Jr

Faster Stronger Wiser Fitness

Cycle Hero

Created by Glenn Payne Jr.

NASM, AFAA Certified Trainer

Precision Nutrition Level 1 Coach

Spartan SGX Coach

For more routines visit

Fasterstrongerwiser.com

This 10-day workout focuses on developing strength and coordination and gives you a new look at cycling workouts.

Sample Calendar						
Mon	**Tues**	**Wed**	**Thurs**	**Fri**	**Sat**	**Sun**
Day 1 Dumbbells	Day 2 Dumbbells 2	Day 3 Resist Bands	Day 4 Weight Plate	Day 5 Barbell	Rest Day 1	Rest Day 2
Day 6 Dumbbells	Day 7 Dumbbells 2	Day 8 Resist Bands	Day 9 Weight Plate	Day 10 Barbell	Rest Day 1	Rest Day 2

Before you get started.

Have a towel and water available because you will sweat a lot. This workout program is also part of The Hero Training Program, a 100-day full-body transformation program.

Disclaimer:

The exercises featured in this workout program are intense, so consult your physician before joining any fitness class or workout hosted by Faster Stronger Wiser Fitness and Glenn Payne Jr.

Faster Stronger Wiser Fitness and Glenn Payne Jr are not responsible for any injuries, sickness, or death from participating in this workout program.

Equipment Needed

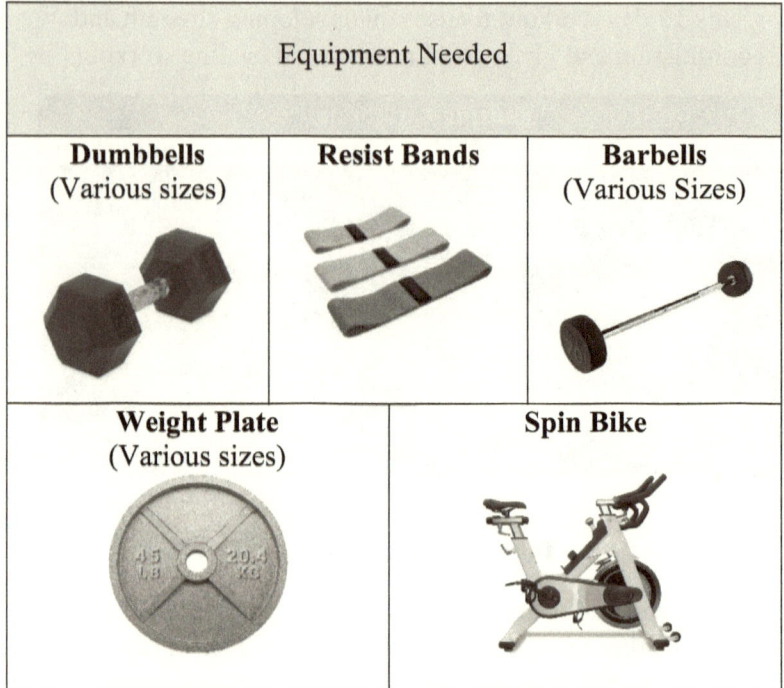

Dumbbells
(Various sizes)

Resist Bands

Barbells
(Various Sizes)

Weight Plate
(Various sizes)

Spin Bike

Table of Contents

How to set up your exercise bike

Start by placing your bike on level ground.

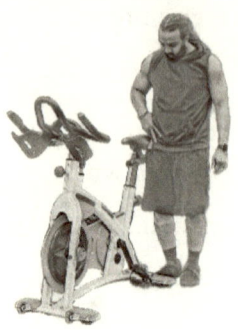

Next, stand next to your bike and put two fingers (pointer and middle) on your hip bone. Your seat should be at the same level as your hip bone. Adjust the seat to that height.

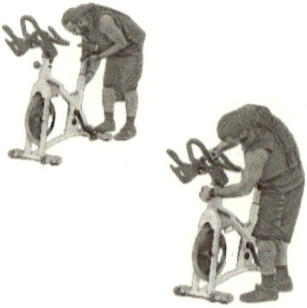

Once your seat is adjusted, ensure it's locked in, then raise the handlebars to an inch higher than your seat.

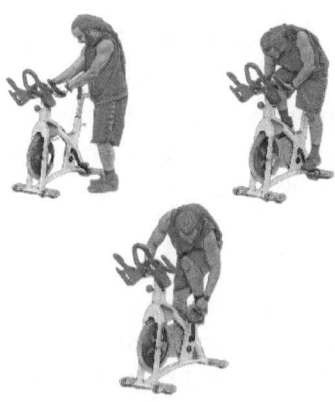

Once your bike is set, climb on and start to pedal. Your knees should NOT lock out as you pedal and should be able to point your toe entirely towards the ground on every rotation.

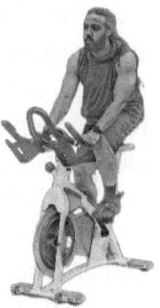

Your hands should be comfortable sitting in front of the handlebars, and your arms should bend slightly in each position.

Cycle Strength, aka. Cycle Hero

The cycle hero exercises do not use reps. Everything is timed to maximize the workout without worrying about counting every repetition. Rest breaks are included in the routine, and the goal is to keep moving the entire time.

Why add weight to the bike?

Cycling workouts have been primarily used for cardiovascular training, and traditional weight training was usually reserved for post-cardio routines. When I first became a cycling instructor in 2016, I wanted to find a way to make cycling classes more exciting. I played around with the different methods, from tossing medicine balls to jump intervals to splitting half of the course into teams and making them compete in speed drills. One day, I was practicing for class and thought, what if you lifted some dumbbells while working on the bike? I decided to grab some dumbbells, and I started performing bicep curls on the bike. In 1 minute, I realized I had worked harder than I would have if I had done the two exercises separately. I immediately came up with a routine and added it to my class. Over the next few years, the combo of weights on the bike became a hit with my students, and to this day, cycling has become one of my most popular classes. The most popular review I would get from this type of workout was that it saved time in the gym because it gave people their cardio and strength workout in under an hour. Many of my members lost weight and developed new types of strength using this workout style; some referred to it as a superhero workout on the bike. That's where the name Cycle Hero came from.

Is the workout safe?

That is one question I received from skeptics when introducing this workout to them, and the answer is yes. When you use weights on the bike, the goal is to go light to ensure you can maintain a comfortable position on the bike as you exercise. You get muscle-building benefits from the amount of time spent on each exercise. Finally, because your legs constantly move, you must maintain good posture to stay balanced on the bike. All these elements combined into one routine make the workout more effective than traditional routines.

Cycle Hero Workout Breakdown

Each routine contains five exercises. Each exercise is performed in a circuit with a 5-minute warmup and cool-down. Every exercise lasts 30 seconds, with a 30-second rest for five rounds. The total runtime of each routine is 35 minutes, which will allow you to incorporate the universal Hero Training Warm Up and Cool Down. In week two of the workout, all time limits will increase to 1 minute, increasing the workout to 60 Minutes plus the warm up and cool down. The increase in time will help you build muscular endurance.

The tempo of every workout runs on the rpm of your feet, which is at two counts (1,2,1,2,1,2). Maintaining this tempo allows you to keep a consistent pace and perform the weighted reps at a consistent 1:0:1 tempo, which means 1 starts the rep, 0 seconds hold, and 1 completes the rep.

Track Your Progress

You will only know if this program works if you track your progress. Five fitness tests will be conducted throughout this program to indicate how your body is progressing visually. Results will vary and can be affected through a solid nutrition regimen. This program does not offer nutrition advice or recommendations.

Use these statistics to track your progress throughout this program to see how your body changes from an aesthetic and performance viewpoint.

Body Statistics: Weight, Body Fat% and Measurements

The Faster Stronger Wiser Fitness Test

As well as the measurements and body fat%, the ability to master your body weight is a testament to your overall fitness level. The Faster Stronger Wiser Fitness test is based on timed bodyweight exercises. The full body weight test is 12 minutes long, and the entire test closes with a 1-mile run for time, which can be done outdoors or on a treadmill.

(Pro tip. Try to use the same running method each time to measure your progress better.)

On the next page, there are three fitness tests. Each one should be completed after completing the full Body Weight Blast Program.

Body Stats

	Test #1 Complete before starting the program.	Test #2 Complete after Week One	Test #3 Complete after Week Two
Date			
Weight			
Body Fat %			
Measurements			
Chest			
Waist			
Hips			
Right Arm			
Left Arm			
Right Leg			
Left Leg			

Fitness Tests

	Test #1 Complete before starting the program.	Test #2 Complete after Week One	Test #3 Complete after Week Two
Date			
Max Push Ups 3 Mins			
Rest 1 Minute			
Max Pull Ups 3 Mins			
Rest 1 Minute			
Max Squats 3 Mins			
Rest 1 Minute			
Max Burpees 3 Mins			
Rest 1 Minute			
1 Mile Run Time			

Faster Stronger Wiser Fitness

Week One

Each day will feel tough because of the time limit associated with each exercise. Focus on maintaining your form throughout each exercise. Take time to complete the warmup and ensure you finish the cool down to complete the workout.

Close your eyes as you perform each exercise to add intensity to the workout.

Rest Days

Use these days to recover for the next week. Take a cold shower for 3-5 minutes daily to reduce your recovery time. This routine will work muscles that you haven't used before.

Day 1: Dumbbells

This workout blends the benefits of both cardiovascular training and strength training. You'll need an exercise bike and a set of dumbbells. Cycling and weightlifting provide a full-body workout targeting various muscle groups while boosting cardiovascular fitness.

Hero Training Warmup (Complete in a circuit)				
	Exercise	**Sets**	**Reps**	**Tempo**
1	Shoulder Tap to Superman	2	10	1:1:1
2	Split Stance Walk Out Combo	2	10	1:1:1

Workout (Complete in a circuit)					
	Exercise	**Sets**	**Reps**	**Tempo**	**Weight**
1	Dumbbell Curls	5	30secs	30secs	
2	Dumbbell Chest Openers	5	30secs	30secs	
3	Dumbbell Shoulder Press	5	30secs	30secs	
4	Dumbbell Row (Right side)	5	30secs	30secs	
5	Dumbbell Row (Left side)	5	30secs	30secs	

Hero Training Cool Down				
	Exercise	**Sets**	**Reps**	**Tempo**
1	Split Stance Walk Out Combo	1	10	1:1:1

Full exercise list and descriptions are available on page 26.

Day 2: Weight Plate

Performing weight plate exercises on an exercise bike is a unique and challenging way to achieve a full-body workout. This full-body workout combines the benefits of cycling with weight plate exercises, providing cardiovascular training and strength conditioning. You'll need an exercise bike and a weight plate.

Hero Training Warmup (Complete in a circuit)				
	Exercise	**Sets**	**Reps**	**Tempo**
1	Shoulder Tap to Superman	2	10	1:1:1
2	Split Stance Walk Out Combo	2	10	1:1:1

Workout (Complete in a circuit)					
	Exercise	**Sets**	**Reps**	**Tempo**	**Weight**
1	Plate Chest Press	5	30secs	30secs	
2	Plate Shoulder Press	5	30secs	30secs	
3	Plate Triceps Extension	5	30secs	30secs	
4	Plate Halos (Right Side)	5	30secs	30secs	
5	Plate Halos (Left Side)	5	30secs	30secs	

Hero Training Cool Down				
	Exercise	**Sets**	**Reps**	**Tempo**
1	Split Stance Walk Out Combo	1	10	1:1:1

Full exercise list and descriptions are available on page 28.

Day 3: Weight Plate Strength

This unique workout blends the benefits of cycling on an exercise bike with weight plate exercises, providing cardiovascular training and full-body strength conditioning. You'll need an exercise bike and a weight plate.

Hero Training Warmup (Complete in a circuit)				
	Exercise	Sets	Reps	Tempo
1	Shoulder Tap to Superman	2	10	1:1:1
2	Split Stance Walk Out Combo	2	10	1:1:1

Workout (Complete in a circuit)				
	Exercise	Sets	Reps	Tempo	Weight
1	Forward Raises	5	30secs	30secs	
2	Steering Wheels	5	30secs	30secs	
3	Plate Flips	5	30secs	30secs	
4	Iso Chest Plate Hold	5	30secs	30secs	
5	Iso Shoulder Plate Hold	5	30secs	30secs	

Hero Training Cool Down				
	Exercise	Sets	Reps	Tempo
1	Split Stance Walk Out Combo	1	10	1:1:1

Full exercise list and descriptions are available on page 30.

Day 4: Resistance Bands

This workout combines the benefits of cycling on an exercise bike with resistance band exercises, providing cardiovascular training and full-body strength conditioning. You'll need an exercise bike and a set of resistance bands.

Hero Training Warmup (Complete in a circuit)				
	Exercise	**Sets**	**Reps**	**Tempo**
1	Shoulder Tap to Superman	2	10	1:1:1
2	Split Stance Walk Out Combo	2	10	1:1:1
Workout (Complete in a circuit)				
	Exercise	**Sets**	**Time**	**Rest**
1	Resist Band Chest Opener	5	30secs	30secs
2	Resist Band Shoulder Opener	5	30secs	30secs
3	Resist Band Circles	5	30secs	30secs
4	Resist Band Chest Opener Hold	5	30secs	30secs
5	Resist Band Shoulder Opener Hold	5	30secs	30secs
Hero Training Cool Down				
	Exercise	**Sets**	**Reps**	**Tempo**
1	Split Stance Walk Out Combo	1	10	1:1:1

Full exercise list and descriptions are available on page 32.

Day 5: Barbells

This workout blends the benefits of both cardiovascular training and strength training. You'll need an exercise bike and a light barbell. The barbell should be light enough to control with one hand and short in length so you won't be thrown off balance while using it on the bike. You can use a weighted stick if you are uncomfortable with a barbell.

Hero Training Warmup (Complete in a circuit)				
	Exercise	Sets	Reps	Tempo
1	Shoulder Tap to Superman	2	10	1:1:1
2	Split Stance Walk Out Combo	2	10	1:1:1
Workout (Complete in a circuit)				
	Exercise	Sets	Reps	Tempo	Weight
1	Chest Press	5	30secs	30secs	
2	Front Shoulder Press	5	30secs	30secs	
3	Back Shoulder Press	5	30secs	30secs	
4	Forward Raise	5	30secs	30secs	
5	Rowers	5	30secs	30secs	
Hero Training Cool Down				
	Exercise	Sets	Reps	Tempo
1	Split Stance Walk Out Combo	1	10	1:1:1

Full exercise list and descriptions are available on page 34.

Week Two

This week focuses on increasing the time limits of the exercises. The goal is to complete each exercise without stopping. Doubling the time used in each routine will push your body past its limits. This process will help you develop more strength and endurance.

Rest Days

Use these days to recover for the next week. Take a cold shower for 3-5 minutes daily to reduce your recovery time. This routine will work muscles that you haven't used before.

Day 6: Dumbbells II

This day repeats day one, but the time is increased to make the workout more challenging.

	Hero Training Warmup (Complete in a circuit)			
	Exercise	**Sets**	**Reps**	**Tempo**
1	Shoulder Tap to Superman	2	10	1:1:1
2	Split Stance Walk Out Combo	2	10	1:1:1

	Workout (Complete in a circuit)				
	Exercise	**Sets**	**Reps**	**Tempo**	**Weight**
1	Dumbbell Curls	5	1min	1min	
2	Dumbbell Chest Openers	5	1min	1min	
3	Dumbbell Shoulder Press	5	1min	1min	
4	Dumbbell Row (Right side)	5	1min	1min	
5	Dumbbell Row (Left side)	5	1min	1min	

	Hero Training Cool Down			
	Exercise	**Sets**	**Reps**	**Tempo**
1	Split Stance Walk Out Combo	1	10	1:1:1

Full exercise list and descriptions are available on page 26.

Day 7: Weight Plate II

This day repeats day two, but the time is increased to make the workout more challenging.

Hero Training Warmup (Complete in a circuit)			
Exercise	**Sets**	**Reps**	**Tempo**
1 Shoulder Tap to Superman	2	10	1:1:1
2 Split Stance Walk Out Combo	2	10	1:1:1

Workout (Complete in a circuit)				
Exercise	**Sets**	**Reps**	**Tempo**	**Weight**
1 Plate Chest Press	5	1min	1min	
2 Plate Shoulder Press	5	1min	1min	
3 Plate Triceps Extension	5	1min	1min	
4 Plate Halos (Right Side)	5	1min	1min	
5 Plate Halos (Left Side)	5	1min	1min	

Hero Training Cool Down			
Exercise	**Sets**	**Reps**	**Tempo**
1 Split Stance Walk Out Combo	1	10	1:1:1

Full exercise list and descriptions are available on page 28.

Day 8: Weight Plate Strength II

This day repeats day three, but the time is increased to make the workout more challenging.

Hero Training Warmup (Complete in a circuit)			
Exercise	Sets	Reps	Tempo
1	Shoulder Tap to Superman	2	10	1:1:1
2	Split Stance Walk Out Combo	2	10	1:1:1

Workout (Complete in a circuit)				
Exercise	Sets	Reps	Tempo	Weight
1	Forward Raises	5	1min	1min	
2	Steering Wheels	5	1min	1min	
3	Plate Flips	5	1min	1min	
4	Iso Chest Plate Hold	5	1min	1min	
5	Iso Shoulder Plate Hold	5	1min	1min	

Hero Training Cool Down			
Exercise	Sets	Reps	Tempo
1	Split Stance Walk Out Combo	1	10	1:1:1

Full exercise list and descriptions are available on page 30.

Day 9: Resistance Bands II

This day repeats day four, but the time is increased to make the workout more challenging.

Hero Training Warmup (Complete in a circuit)			
	Exercise	**Sets**	**Reps**	**Tempo**
1	Shoulder Tap to Superman	2	10	1:1:1
2	Split Stance Walk Out Combo	2	10	1:1:1
Workout (Complete in a circuit)			
	Exercise	**Sets**	**Time**	**Rest**
1	Resist Band Chest Opener	5	1min	1min
2	Resist Band Shoulder Opener	5	1min	1min
3	Resist Band Circles	5	1min	1min
4	Resist Band Chest Opener Hold	5	1min	1min
5	Resist Band Shoulder Opener Hold	5	1min	1min
Hero Training Cool Down			
	Exercise	**Sets**	**Reps**	**Tempo**
1	Split Stance Walk Out Combo	1	10	1:1:1

Full exercise list and descriptions are available on page 32.

Faster Stronger Wiser Fitness

Day 10: Barbells II

This day repeats day five, but the time is increased to make the workout more challenging.

Hero Training Warmup (Complete in a circuit)			
Exercise	**Sets**	**Reps**	**Tempo**
1 Shoulder Tap to Superman	2	10	1:1:1
2 Split Stance Walk Out Combo	2	10	1:1:1

Workout (Complete in a circuit)				
Exercise	**Sets**	**Reps**	**Tempo**	**Weight**
1 Chest Press	5	1min	1min	
2 Front Shoulder Press	5	1min	1min	
3 Back Shoulder Press	5	1min	1min	
4 Forward Raise	5	1min	1min	
5 Rowers	5	1min	1min	

Hero Training Cool Down			
Exercise	**Sets**	**Reps**	**Tempo**
1 Split Stance Walk Out Combo	1	10	1:1:1

Full exercise list and descriptions are available on page 34.

Cycle Hero Exercise List
Hero Training Warmup & Cool Down

Shoulder Taps to Superman

Start in a plank position with your hands under your shoulders and your feet hip-width apart. Tap your shoulders with each hand, then lower yourself to the ground. Next, extend your arms in front of your body and lift your chest, arms, and legs off the ground as if you were flying. Return to the plank position.

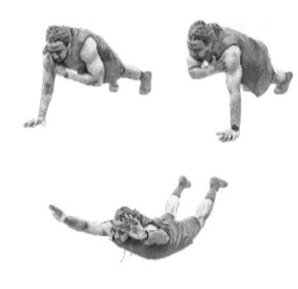

Split Stance Walk Out Combo

Start with your feet in a split stance. Next, bend forward until your hands touch the ground. Walk your hands out until you are in a cobra stretch. Focus on pressing your hips into the ground for 3 seconds. Next, release the stretch and touch your toes, going right hand to left toe and left hand to right toe. Return to the starting point.

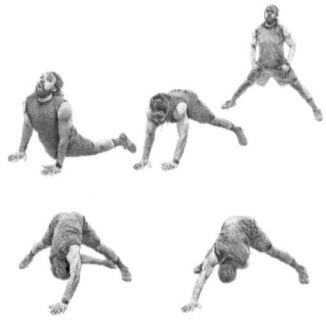

Day 1: Dumbbells

Dumbbell Curls
Start on the bike, in the seat, at a comfortable resistance. Grab a dumbbell in each hand, and then perform a bicep curl. Keep your chest up.

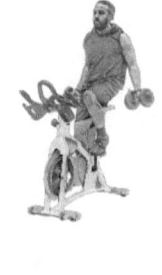 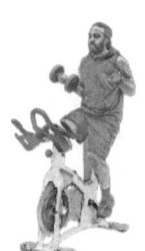

Dumbbell Shoulder Press
Start on the bike, in the seat, at a comfortable resistance. Grab a dumbbell in each hand, stack the dumbbells on your shoulder, then perform a shoulder press.

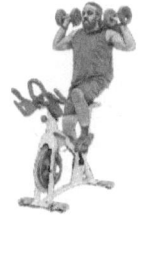 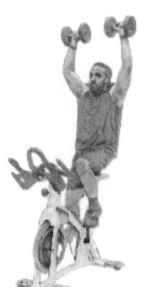

Dumbbell Chest Openers
Start on the bike, in the seat, at a comfortable resistance. Grab a dumbbell in each hand and hold them in an underhand grip at chest level. Widen out your arms, then bring them back together.

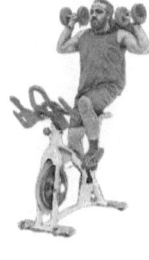 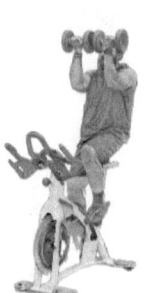

Dumbbell Rows

Start on the bike, out of the seat, at a heavy resistance to maintain balance. Place one arm over the handlebars, flatten your back, and push your hips over the seat. Hold a dumbbell in your opposite hand and pull the dumbbell up to your ribs. Repeat the exercise on the opposite side.

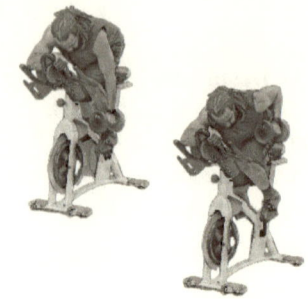

Day 2: Weight Plate

Plate Chest Press

Start on the bike, in the seat, at a comfortable resistance. Hold a weighted plate at chest level. Press the plate out in front of you. Keep your chest up.

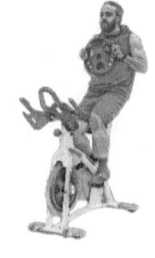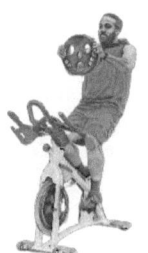

Plate Shoulder Press

Start on the bike, in the seat, at a comfortable resistance. Grab a weighted plate, hold it at chest level, and press it above your head. Keep your chest up.

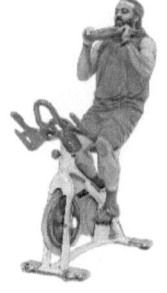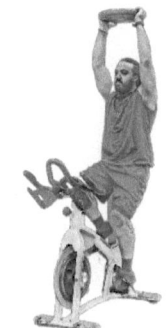

Plate Triceps Extension

Start on the bike, in the seat, at a comfortable resistance. Grab a weighted plate and hold it above your head. Lower the weight behind your head, then extend it back up. Keep your chest up.

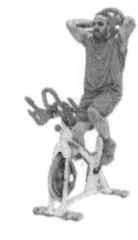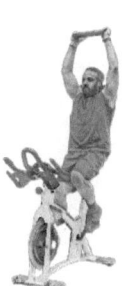

Plate Halos

Start on the bike, in the seat, at a comfortable resistance. Grab a weighted plate and hold it above your head. Wrap the weight around your head in a circular motion. Try to keep it as close to your head as possible. Repeat on the opposite side.

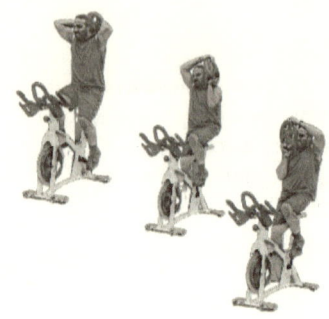

Day 3: Weight Plate Strength

Forward Raises

Start on the bike, in the seat, at a comfortable resistance. Hold a weighted plate at chest level. Raise the weight above your head and return it to the starting point.

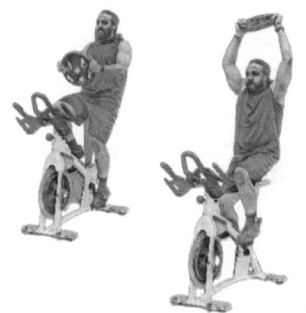

Steering Wheels

Start on the bike, in the seat, at a comfortable resistance. Hold a weighted plate at chest level. Rotate the plate as if you are turning a steering wheel. Repeat the motion.

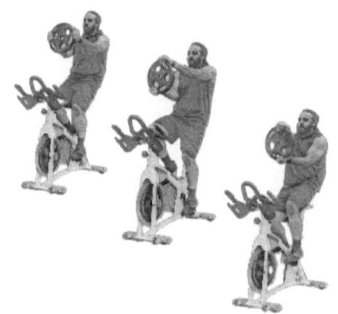

Plate Flips

Start on the bike, in the seat, at a comfortable resistance. Hold a weighted plate at chest level. Turn the plate vertically as if you are flipping the plate over.

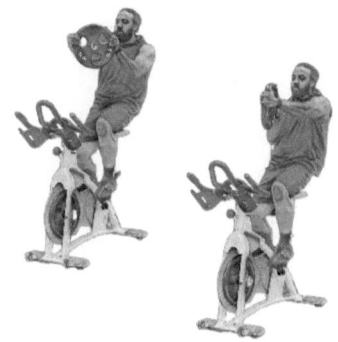

Iso Chest Plate Hold

Start on the bike, in the seat, at a comfortable resistance. Hold a weighted plate at chest level. Hold that position.

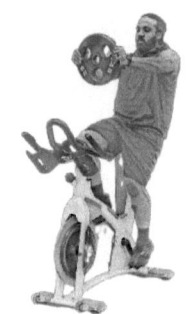

Iso Shoulder Plate Hold

Start on the bike, in the seat, at a comfortable resistance. Hold a weighted plate above your head. Hold that position.

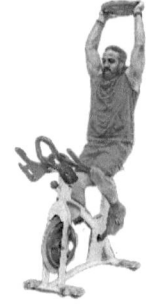

Day 4: Resistance Bands

Resist Band Chest Opener

Start on the bike, in the seat, at a comfortable resistance. Place a resistance band around your forearms and hold them at chest level. Widen your arms as far as possible and return them to the starting position.

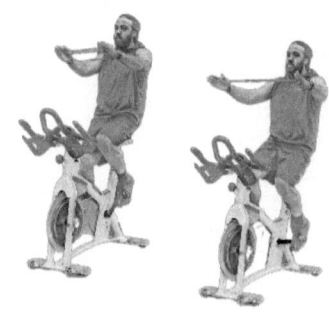

Resist Band Shoulder Opener

Start on the bike, in the seat, at a comfortable resistance. Place a resistance band around your forearms and hold them above your head. Widen your arms as far as possible and return them to the starting position.

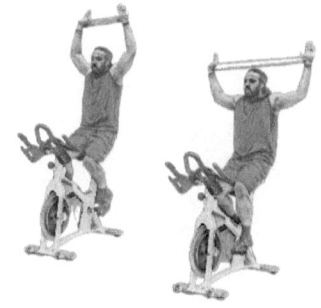

Resist Band Circles

Start on the bike, in the seat, at a comfortable resistance. Place a resistance band around your forearms and hold them at chest level. Rotate your arms in a circular motion. Widen your arms as far as possible and return them to the starting position.

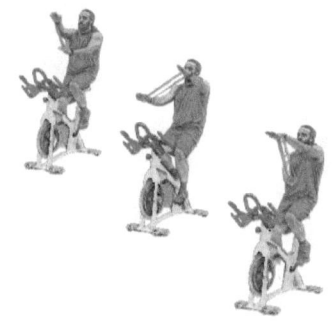

Resist Band Chest Opener Hold

Start on the bike, in the seat, at a comfortable resistance. Place a resistance band around your forearms and hold them at chest level. Widen out your arms as far as you can and hold that position.

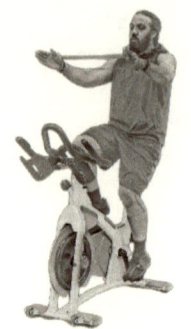

Resist Band Shoulder Opener Hold

Start on the bike, in the seat, at a comfortable resistance. Place a resistance band around your forearms and hold them above your head. Widen out your arms as far as you can and hold that position.

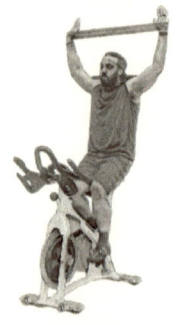

Day 5: Barbells

Chest Press

Start on the bike, in the seat, at a comfortable resistance. Hold a barbell at chest level. Pull the barbell back to your chest and press it back to the starting point.

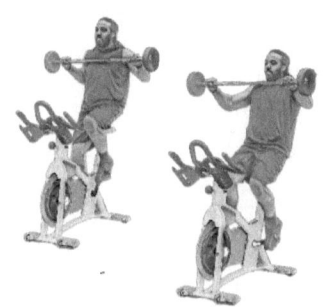

Front Shoulder Press

Start on the bike, in the seat, at a comfortable resistance. Grab a barbell, hold it at the top of your chest, and press it above your head. Keep your chest up.

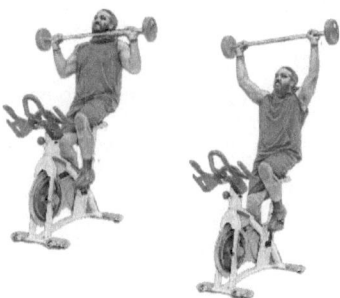

Back Shoulder Press

Start on the bike, in the seat, at a comfortable resistance. Grab a barbell, hold it behind your back, and press it above your head. Keep your chest up.

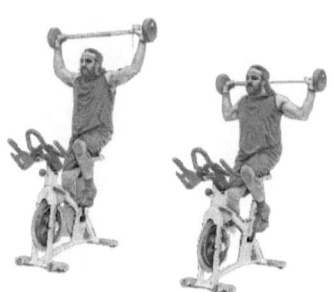

Forward Raise

Start on the bike, in the seat, at a comfortable resistance. Hold a barbell at chest level. Raise the barbell above your head and return it to the starting point.

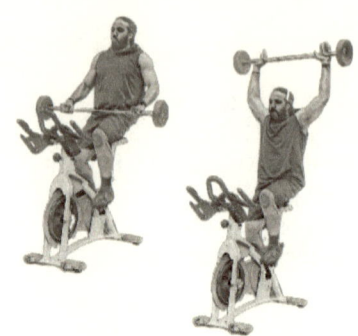

Rowers

Start on the bike, in the seat, at a comfortable resistance. Hold a barbell at chest level. Rotate the barbell as if you are rowing in a rowboat. Repeat the motion.

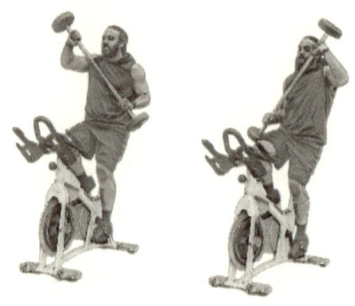

Thank You

Thank you for challenging yourself with this workout program.
This is one portion of the FSW Hero Training Program.

www.ingramcontent.com/pod-product-compliance
Lightning Source LLC
Chambersburg PA
CBHW020332290526
45785CB00007B/3029